**The Medical
Job Interview**

# The Medical Job Interview
## Secrets for Success

Colin J. Mumford

BMedSci, BM, BS, DM, FRCP, FRCPEdin, Dip IMC RCSEd
Consultant Neurologist
Department of Clinical Neurosciences
Western General Hospital
Edinburgh

**SECOND EDITION**

**Blackwell**
Publishing

Published by Blackwell Publishing Ltd

Blackwell Publishing, Inc., 350 Main Street, Malden, Massachusetts 02148-5020, USA

Blackwell Publishing Ltd, 9600 Garsington Road, Oxford OX4 2DQ, UK

Blackwell Publishing Asia Pty Ltd, 550 Swanston Street, Carlton, Victoria 3053, Australia

First published 2000
Second edition 2005
3      2006

Library of Congress Cataloging-in-Publication Data

Mumford, Colin John.
   The medical job interview : secrets for success / Colin John Mumford. —2nd ed.
      p. ; cm.
   Includes bibliographical references and index.
   ISBN 13. 978-1-4051-2185-9
   ISBN 1-4051-2185-8 (alk. paper)
   1. Medicine—Vocational guidance—Great Britain.   2. Employment
interviewing—Great Britain.   3. Physicians—Employment—Great Britain.
   [DNLM:   1. Interviews.   2. Job Application.   3. Physicians.   W 21 M962m
2005]   I. Title.

   R690.M785 2005
   610.69′0941—dc22

                                                                              2004021461

ISBN-13: 978-1-4051-2185-9
ISBN-10: 1-4051-2185-8

A catalogue record for this title is available from the British Library

Set in 9/12 pt Palatino by SNP Best-set Typesetter Ltd., Hong Kong
Printed and bound in India by Replika Press Pvt., Ltd

Commissioning Editor: Vicki Noyes
Editorial Assistant: Nic Ulyatt
Development Editors: Lorna Hind, Mirjana Misina
Production Controller: Kate Charman

For further information on Blackwell Publishing, visit our website:
http://www.blackwellpublishing.com

# CONTENTS

# PREFACE TO THE SECOND EDITION

I was a bit surprised by the success of the first edition of this book. People whom I'd never met came up to me in corridors and at medical meetings and asked me whether I was the author. Most of them expressed gratitude for the book, and one or two were positively effusive in their thanks. Such comments have been most welcome and sometimes rather embarrassing.

A few individuals, usually senior medical staff who have entered the murky world of hospital management, were less convinced of the book's value. Some suggested that it provided an incentive for junior hospital doctors somehow to 'cheat' or to 'gain an unfair advantage'. One medical director of a major district general hospital took the trouble to write to me to suggest that some aspects of the contents were possibly unlawful and recommended 'inappropriate practice'.

I have to say that I think these individuals have misunderstood the purpose of this book. My goal in writing it was not to present any sort of overview of the 'official constitution' of the interview process for doctors advancing their medical careers. Rather my aim was to draw together a selection of 'tips and tricks' specifically aimed at those junior doctors who might feel at a disadvantage compared with their colleagues when faced with a medical job interview, in order to help themselves to a greater degree of success.

I will leave it to the reader to decide if I've got it right.

# ACKNOWLEDGEMENTS

A large number of good friends have helped me in the preparation of this second edition. Suggestions for new content, and comments on old, have come from senior hospital doctors, junior doctors in training, secondary school teachers, representatives of the pharmaceutical industry and members of some of the more interesting parts of the British Civil Service. To all of these people I would like to offer enormous thanks.

# NOTE FOR WOULD-BE MEDICAL STUDENTS

This book is written for final-year medical students and junior hospital doctors in training. It is not really intended to be a guide to help sixth-formers who are seeking a place at medical school. Nevertheless, I know that a number of copies of the first edition have been sold to A-level candidates, and I suspect some of the suggestions that I have made are applicable to the process of gaining entry into university. Certainly, I think some of the ideas regarding 'pre-interview groundwork' could be utilised by the enthusiastic sixth-former wanting to make sure that they receive a good offer from their first-choice medical school.

# INTRODUCTION

## chapter 1

The aim of this short book is simple. It is to make you successful in your next medical job interview. It is quite possible to be a wonderful medical student or doctor with encyclopaedic knowledge of medical conditions, first-class clinical skills and a terrific rapport with all your patients, but if you can't perform well in the job interviews then you will get nowhere. This book sets out to give you tips that will be equally relevant, whether you are a final-year medical student applying for your first house job, a senior house officer (SHO) trying to break through on to the specialist registrar career ladder, or if you are reaching the end of your specialist registrar training and are seeking appointment to your first consultant post.

Note that virtually all that is contained in this book is relevant to the UK system of medical training. Graduates in Ireland and Western Europe may find some of the information given useful. I must leave it up to colleagues in the USA and Canada to decide whether they feel that this 'very British approach' can win over interview panels in North America!

Even British graduates need to appreciate that I am giving advice from the point of view of a hospital consultant who has worked his way up through the British *hospital* medical career ladder. A rather different emphasis and series of tricks are needed in breaking into the world of general practice. All the same, some of the tips that I give here may at least be starters for someone approaching an interview to be a registrar in general practice, or even seeking appointment to their first post as principal in general practice.

The astonishing thing about most British medical graduates is that although they prepare in enormous detail for clinical medical school exams and for postgraduate diplomas, such as the MRCP(UK), MRCOG, FRCS and so on, most of them put relatively little thought into planning their strategy for handling a medical job interview. This is a grave error since there is no doubt that good interview technique can be learned. Some people begin their careers already good at it, but others are so bad they could be described as appalling in an interview, and it is this latter group who most need to do their homework prior to facing an interview panel!

Throughout this book I've tended to use the word 'he' when, of course, I mean 'he or she'. Writing 'he or she' every time becomes clumsy.

# BEFORE THE INTERVIEW

## chapter 2

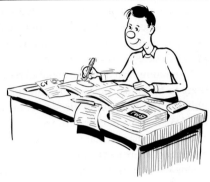

## SPOTTING THE ADVERT

It sounds ridiculous, but some individuals fail at the very first hurdle in their efforts to climb the medical career ladder and that is because they fail to spot the advert for the job which they want. This is a catastrophic mistake since the one way to guarantee not being short listed is not to apply for the job in the first place. Therefore, as soon as you are even contemplating applying for your next move up the medical ladder you should be scrutinising the relevant medical press to see which adverts are appearing, what sort of jobs are available and starting to focus your mind on the places where you would most like to work. This may mean remaining in your own geographical area, or you may have a particular desire to move to a different part of the country for your next job.

In general terms this task is made easy for British graduates because the classified section of the *British Medical Journal* lists all the available jobs coming up, and these are conveniently grouped under headings according to speciality. Remember, however, that editors and typesetters of the *British Medical Journal* are human, and it is not uncommon to see an advert for a post, say, in neurology, advertised in error under the section headed neurosurgery. Occasionally, hospitals perform rather underhand tricks, and — for reasons best known to themselves — may decide to place an advert in a not-very-obvious location, which may be in a national newspaper, in the back pages of a weekly free journal such as *Hospital Doctor* or in some other obscure site.

If you think that a post is about to be advertised yet are struggling to find the actual advertisement, then there is no harm in phoning the appropriate personnel or medical staffing department at the relevant hospital or regional postgraduate centre and asking when a particular post will be coming up. Expressing such enthusiasm at an early stage does no harm at all.

One word of caution is required at this point, and that is this: some individuals are uncertain whether or not they should apply for a job. This is particularly true at the start of a medical career when people are not sure if they should hold out for 'the best' pre-registration house officer job or whether they should accept something 'second-rate'. Equally, this is especially acute at the end of the medical ladder when senior specialist registrars are uncertain whether a 'plum consultant post' is about to come up or whether they should go for a post which they might consider 'second division'. The way to decide whether to apply or not is that if you eventually get through to the medical interview and find yourself successful, you need to ask: 'Will I stand up, punch the air and shout "Yahooo!" if I am successful?' If you are uncertain as to whether you would be able to express such overt enthusiasm then probably you should not be applying for the post at all. This rule is there to be broken, however, and if you are genuinely not sure whether a job is the right one for you then there is no harm in putting in an application and at least going part-way through the selection process, provided that you withdraw before you find yourself sitting in the interview. You can withdraw, if necessary, on the morning of the interview but it is a complete no–no to sit in an interview, be offered the job and then reject the offer following the interview. This goes down extremely badly with interview panels and will land you with an undesirable reputation. On the other hand, a cautious application and polite, tactful withdrawal prior to the interview, with careful explanation to the relevant consultants, will not usually cause too much upset.

## 'THE COMMANDO OPERATION' TO GET ON THE SHORT LIST

Once you have seen the correct advert for you then the next steps, which include submitting the application, preparing your curriculum vitae (CV) and making sure you get on the short list, can best be thought of as a 'commando operation'. Royal Marine commandos are enormously successful at what they do basically because they leave no margin for error. Every item of equipment is checked, rechecked and tested in enormous detail. If you seriously want to be successful in the medical job interview then you need to begin a thorough, almost military, operation to make absolutely sure that you get the job. Like it or not, job interviews are competitive and accordingly you have to show the interview panel that you are better than everybody else that has made an application for the post. Since some jobs may receive in excess of 200 applicants, then if you sit back and wait to be short-listed you can guarantee that you will simply be a 'face in the crowd' and you are very unlikely to be short-listed unless there is something extraordinarily unusual about your CV.

Therefore, as soon as the appropriate job advert appears you need to be on the phone to get the relevant application forms and you need to start preparing your CV. The application forms will almost certainly give you information about the hospital, including names of relevant consultants and appropriate contact phone numbers.

Your immediate goal following receipt of the job description is to get yourself onto the short list. Other people can help you with this. Indeed, a well-judged phone call from one of your current consultants to his friend or golfing partner, who is a consultant in the relevant hospital, can work wonders. You may feel that this is somehow underhand in asking your consultant to make a phone call on your behalf, but, unfortunately, some of your competitors will have done this, and you need to make sure you are playing in the same ball game. Bear in mind that although a helpful phone call putting forward your name may significantly improve your chances of getting on to the short list, once you are on the short list you are on your own and it is very unlikely that persuasive words from one of your senior colleagues will actually make a difference in the interview itself.

## TO VISIT OR NOT TO VISIT?

Many candidates wonder if it is 'worthwhile' visiting the relevant hospital before the short list is announced. Anybody who does not visit the hospital is, in my view, significantly reducing their chance of getting placed on the short list. There is no doubt that a voluntary visit, made early, and made at your own expense in order to look around wards, departments, x-ray facilities, and so on—and ideally to meet one or two of the consultants—can be enormously rewarding. The progress of a whole career can be changed by 'bumping into' the relevant consultant or professor in the corridor outside his office. If you can achieve this then you are already one rung higher than all your competitors in the fight to get on to the short list. Be mindful of the fact that most senior consultants are very busy and do not take kindly to being interrupted in their office or being stopped whilst walking in the corridor outside their office. Therefore, you need to be sharp and to the point in introducing yourself to them and asking if there is a point 'later in the day' when you might be able to spend 5 minutes with them since you are 'most interested' in the forthcoming job on their unit. Most consultants will accept this sort of approach but will not wish to spend 5 or 10 minutes in the corridor discussing things when they, undoubtedly, will have more important things to do.

However, a request to meet later in the day may be acceptable to them.

If, having 'bumped into' the relevant consultant, you find he is still not willing to see you, then there is no reason at all why you should not go and see his secretary and ask if you might talk to him on another occasion, or whether there are a few moments at the end of the day when he will be less busy. If nothing else you can attempt to endear yourself to the relevant secretary such that she may make a favourable comment later in the day when she is dealing with other aspects of the consultant's work.

This initial visit must not be confused with the visits that are frequently made following the publication of the short list. Many hospitals send a letter with their initial information pack saying something to the extent of 'shortlisted candidates are invited to visit the hospital.' These visits will often be arranged and timetabled by the secretary of the most senior consultant involved and the hospital will reimburse you with the costs of your travel. Bear in mind that you will only have the chance of doing this once you are already on the short list, and therefore a visit prior to short-listing is, in my opinion, essential to show enthusiasm and to start to set yourself apart from the crowd.

The process of short-listing will usually be done by the head of the relevant department to which you are applying and also by a number of his consultant colleagues. It is very unlikely that members of the hospital management will be involved in the short-listing process, although occasionally representatives of the regional postgraduate dean may have some votes in this process. Therefore, if you are going to make a visit prior to short-listing, and I advise that you do, then concentrate solely on seeing the clinicians for whom you will be working. If the post which you are applying for is at junior house officer (JHO) or senior house officer (SHO) level, then try to see some of the specialist registrars working on the unit as well, since you would be surprised how much exchange of ideas takes place at the end of a ward round when consultants are discussing with their registrars potential candidates for short-listing.

Although the initial visit that I am advising prior to short-listing could be considered as being 'relatively informal' you need all the while to be aware of the fact that you have one goal only, and that is to convince the people whom you meet that you are the single best candidate for the forthcoming job. Accordingly, part of the process requires that you look smart, engage in appropriately focused conversation with the doctors you meet, and, above all, have a large number of spare copies of your CV to distribute. Most of the senior clinicians will not see your CV until very shortly before they are asked to produce a short list, and so, if your name is to be remembered, you must pull a CV out of your bag and leave it with the relevant consultant 'for his perusal once you are gone.'

Once you have returned to your base hospital following this pre-short-listing visit, make sure that you discuss what went on with your current bosses since if they have not already telephoned their colleagues at the new hospital to put in a word on your behalf, this is the time at which you should ask them to do so.

## WHOM TO SEE ONCE YOU ARE SHORT LISTED?

Once the short list has been produced, and, hopefully, has your name on it, then whether or not you previously visited, you are now absolutely obliged to go and visit the relevant hospital. In general terms your travel expenses for a visit at this stage will be refunded to you. Your priority, once again, is to meet with the consultants for whom you will be working, or, if a senior post, whom you will be working alongside, but bear in mind that during the interview itself there will almost certainly be some non-medical interviewers, e.g. a member of the hospital management or a representative of the Trust Board. Therefore, at least one of your visits must be to the chief executive of the hospital, or, if he is not available, one of his senior management team. The reason for this is that you must be briefed regarding forthcoming developments in the hospital, be they new buildings, new clinics or a new approach to the delivery of medical care to the local community. You can gain a great deal of information by talking to senior managers, and much of this information may not be known to the consultant staff who will be interviewing you. Having learned top quality and up-to-date information from the managers, you can sound highly impressive by discussing the way in which the hospital is going to evolve during the next few years and how you feel that you, as SHO, specialist registrar or consultant, will contribute to 'this blossoming service'. Additionally, and particularly if you are applying for a post at relatively senior level, make sure that you meet one or two consultants from related specialities. So, for example, if you are going for a post in cardiology then ensure you meet some of the cardiac surgeons. If you are applying for a post as a transplant surgeon, then the medical nephrologists and hepatologists would almost certainly be flattered if you took the trouble to meet them prior to the interview. Do not underestimate how much potential candidates are discussed over the table in the consultants' dining room and if your name is mentioned favourably here, it can work wonders in the final reckoning.

If you are struggling to meet the relevant consultants and senior members of the hospital management team, then consider trying to track down the president of the junior doctors' mess. The mess president is very likely to be able to give you up-to-date information regarding what is good and what is bad about the hospital. He may be able to introduce you to SHOs and specialist registrars in the department to which you are applying; all of whom could be very useful sources of information and conversation with them could result in you appearing far better informed than your competitors in the eventual job interview.

## HOW TO CHOOSE A WINNING REFEREE

Selection of referees is not as immediately simple as it might seem. Your priority must be to get people that will say nice things about you. However, some referees are all too willing to give a reference that is remarkably mediocre and does not make you stand out in comparison with the competition. Therefore, you need to go and speak to your potential referees and be prepared to ask them outright if they would be willing to write a *good* reference for you. This may seem to be a rather pushy approach, but there is no doubt that some senior medical staff will willingly agree to be a referee and then write rather uninspired comments which look bad when it comes to the interview. Short matter-of-fact references never help anybody. So feel free to ask your potential referee if they would be willing to write a detailed reference, outlining your good points and explaining the reasons why you would be very suitable for the post which you are proposing to apply for. Also do not hesitate about choosing a larger number of referees than was specifically requested in the job description and advertisement. I advise people that if the request is for two references then the names of three referees should be given. If the request is for three referees then four names should be offered. One reason for this is that hospitals may request references at very short notice and sometimes referees are away or abroad. Failure to produce a reference is a total catastrophe. You must, therefore, offer the names of 'stand-by' referees. Moreover, many personnel departments will simply seek a reference from all of the names given as potential referees without thinking how many they originally specified. If an interview panel is deluged with a large number of strongly worded, glowing references speaking about you in the highest possible terms, then this can do nothing but good.

# GETTING THE CURRICULUM VITAE RIGHT

## chapter 3

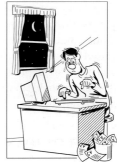

## PRESENTATION

Entire books are devoted to the right and wrong way to present a curriculum vitae (CV), (sometimes called a 'resumé' by our colleagues in North America). Many formats are acceptable, but the document that is presented must look pristine. It must be laser printed and laid out in a simple, readily accessible format. Make sure that the typing is broadly spaced, and that dates describing the time spent in previous posts are clearly laid out. Modern interview panels take great pains to ensure that candidates have done the appropriate amount of general professional training and specialist training, and this is usually done right at the start of the interview. Watching a member of the interview panel struggling to piece together information from a poorly set out CV is desperately embarrassing and generally means rapid failure for the guilty candidate.

## PROFESSIONAL COMPANY?

The back pages of the *British Medical Journal* are now awash with advertisements for professional companies who offer to present your CV in a 'better format'. Unless you are absolutely confident that you have achieved the optimal presentation of your own CV, then it may be worth employing the services of one of these companies. Provided you can afford it, send off your CV, pay the money, and see what they produce. You may be pleasantly surprised to see how much improvement these companies can make, and if you are impressed with the new-look of your own CV then it is very probable that those individuals making the short list will also be impressed.

## ORDER OF JOBS

Most medical CVs are set out in a certain order, usually starting with personal details, education, medical degrees, medical diplomas and higher qualifications, as well as noting registration with the General Medical Council (provisional, full or limited) and membership of a defence organisation. The CV should then describe your present and previous occupations. Unfortunately, this latter point is not as immediately simple as it sounds. Senior medical staff, and probably medical personnel departments as well, seem to be divided into two camps: those that like to see your present job first, with previous posts presented in reverse chronological order, and those that prefer your CV to read like a story book with your junior house officer (JHO) posts first, then senior house officer (SHO) posts, registrar posts and so on. Passions run surprisingly high in this area, but there is very little that you, as the interview candidate, can do in terms of 'mind reading' what the short listers will prefer. My own opinion is that interview panels are generally most interested in what you're doing *now*, and rather less interested in what you have done in the past. Therefore, I would advise going for the reverse chronological order approach, but be aware that it may slightly irritate some people.

Remember to make your present appointment sound as attractive as possible. For example, you may think that you are simply 'specialist registrar in general medicine', but if you think care-fully you might find that you are also an honorary lecturer in medicine of the relevant university or at least a clinical tutor to one or more medical students. All of these facets of your present appointment should be clearly stated.

## GAPS ON THE CV

When describing previous appointments, make sure, above all, that the dates between which each post was held are clearly set out. List the names of the consultants for whom you worked. If you have performed locum posts try to fit these in, in chronological order. In recent years the length of postgraduate training between JHO and consultant posts in medical specialities has tended to shorten, and it has become increasingly important that interview panels are completely certain that all the training requirements needed for appointment to a given post have been completed.

Unexpected gaps in the sequence of jobs in your CV will lead to confusion, and this is to be avoided during the interview. If there are any periods of time in your CV which are unaccounted for, then be certain that you have included a comment to explain what you did during that vacant period. Even if this was time spent in an activity which you feel would not enhance your medical career then you should still include an explanation. Mysterious blanks trouble interview panels. Some candidates nowadays consider presenting their CV with a sort of 'time-line' down the right-hand margin of the pages which detail their career progress, so making it easier for interview panels to follow exactly what they have done since qualification; and this is a good idea.

## OTHER CONTENT

Once you have dealt with present and previous posts in your CV then most interview panels like to see short sections describing your experience in your chosen speciality, teaching experience, management experience and, of course, a detailed description of research and audit work that you have done. You may wish to include a section listing courses and conferences attended. If you are applying for a relatively senior post it is likely that you will have a number of publications and these should be presented in detail. Traditionally, published work is presented in the following order:

books;

chapters in books;

refereed papers;

review articles;

invited editorials;

published abstracts of communications to learned societies;

published correspondence;

poster presentations; and, finally,

any non-medical publications which you may have.

You should conclude your CV by incorporating a section on your career development aims, other relevant information, for example languages spoken and information technology skills, and a short section on your interests and hobbies. The final page should be a list of referees.

## 'DANGEROUS' CV CONTENT

It is difficult to imagine that anything you include in your CV might unintentionally threaten your success in the interview. Nevertheless, it is possible to put things in your CV which might be better left out. Most frequently this problem arises with your list of 'hobbies and interests'. I would urge great caution before going into any detail regarding your membership of political organisations, and also beware of listing your enthusiasm for other groups which may seem innocuous to you, but which might not find favour with some of the more conservative members of the interview panel.

Everyone would agree that it would be foolhardy to list membership of an extremist or violent political organisation your CV, but I was once alarmed to hear that a member of an interview panel drew the attention of a candidate to the fact that he had placed 'member of Amnesty International' under his interests. The interviewee was then asked whether he thought that this was a 'suitable thing' to place in a medical CV. Most of us would be horrified that such a question was asked, and the candidate apparently handled the issue extremely well, but this illustrates the fact, however, that some thought is required regarding the presentation of your interests, since you can never account for unpredictable political leanings of the panel.

## CONTACT DETAILS FOR YOUR REFEREES

The final page of your CV will be a list of your referees. I have already suggested that you should offer the names of one or two more referees than were originally asked for in the job specification. You *must* give comprehensive contact details for all your referees, since human resources departments have a very bad habit of seeking references for candidates only on the morning of the interview, or possibly no more than 1 or 2 days beforehand. Very frequently these departments leave it too late to approach the relevant referee by mail, and they then cannot track them down by phone, so contact by fax or e-mail can sometimes save the day.

So, remember to make sure that you give the correct phone numbers (both direct line and hospital switchboard), the fax number and also the e-mail address for each of your referees, since details about you might well be requested at very short notice.

One final observation is required regarding your CV: do not take it for granted that the main 'selling point' which features in your CV will automatically come out during the interview. It may well be overlooked, and therefore it is up to you to make certain that the interview panel takes notice. Do not assume that they've read something; you need to say it!

# THE INTERVIEW

## chapter 4

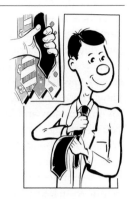

## WHERE, WHEN AND HOW?

If you have followed the instructions in the first part of this book then with luck you will have made it to the short list, and accordingly you will be invited to attend for interview. Like so many aspects of getting on in a medical career, preparation for the interview needs to start even before you receive the letter inviting you to attend. Remember that you are not such an important candidate that the date, time or location of the interview will be changed just to suit you. Therefore, it is perfectly reasonable, when applying for a job, to ask the hospital personnel department if a date has already been set for the interview, and you should ensure that you are not on holiday or out of the country for another reason on the allotted date. Only under very exceptional circumstances will you be able to persuade an interview panel to change the date of an interview, and this is only likely to happen for very senior appointments if you are clearly the front-running candidate.

The second vital issue, which sounds obvious but which is frequently a stumbling block for junior doctors, is the need to find out the exact location of the interview. This is not as simple as it may seem since frequently candidates assume that the interview will take place in the hospital at which they have applied for a job, whereas in fact the interview is held at the regional postgraduate centre, the Trust Board offices or the headquarters of the regional health authority. All these are traps for the unwary, and if this sort of elementary information is not sorted out at an early stage you will be rattled if you eventually do make it to the interview. There is nothing worse than turning up a few minutes late for an interview and having to apologise for being late because you went to the wrong venue. Under no circumstances whatsoever should you be late for the interview since to turn up late implies a degree of shoddy planning which will immediately alienate most senior doctors, who will think that if you are incapable of getting to an interview on time, then there is no chance at all that you will actually make it to their clinic or to their ward rounds on time.

It is perfectly reasonable to try to find out who will be interviewing you. Sometimes for posts at junior house officer (JHO) or senior house officer (SHO) level this may be a panel as small as two individuals. More frequently the panel is much larger than that, and for most specialist registrar appointments, and certainly for consultant grade appointments, the panel may be as big as 11 or 12 people. The reason for this is that most interview panels are now convened to a relatively set formula. There will be some of the consultants for whom you are going to be working, of course, but in addition, there will be representatives of the relevant university, somebody representing the regional postgraduate dean, and a member of the hospital Trust Board. Bear in mind that this latter individual may know very little about medicine and, indeed, may know little about the day-to-day workings of a hospital. This individual is sometimes jokingly referred to using the generic term, 'the vicar's wife'. This person may ask some very unexpected questions, and it is worth being well prepared for the questions that may come from 'the vicar's wife', about which more later.

Note also that for specialist registrar and consultant appointments there will be another important individual who is the Royal College representative, sometimes referred to as the 'national panellist' for interviews in Scotland. This member of the panel has a slightly different remit, in that he is not there to assess who is best for the job, but to ensure that every candidate who attends the interview has done the required amount of previous training, for example general professional training before specialisation, and he also confirms with the chairman of the interview panel that you are 'suitable for appointment to the offered post'.

Remember also that although you may have spent many hours trying to 'bump into' the professor and head of department in the corridor outside his office, whilst he will almost certainly be on the panel, he will not usually be the chairman. The chairman of large interview panels is frequently a consultant from a different speciality and sometimes from a different hospital. Alternatively, this person may be the medical director of the hospital in which you are applying to work. The chairman of the panel is there to ensure fair play and may not, in fact, have a vote in the final judgement as to who is appointed.

Knowing the individual members of the panel in advance can be enormously helpful in being successful in the medical job interview. Once you have heard that you are short listed, you should contact the relevant personnel department and ask if they are able to let you know the composition of the panel. Some hospitals are rather cagey about this, believing it is somehow 'unfair', but in general terms most personnel departments are willing to give you a list and job titles of the people comprising the panel. You should then find out exactly who they are, where they work and what they do. If you have not already met them on a previous visit then you may wish to make a further visit to ensure that your face is known to as many members of the panel as possible.

The interview itself is likely to be held in a large, relatively formal, room. Many hospitals have a 'board room' which they reserve almost exclusively for this purpose. In the same way that you must know exactly the geographical location of the interview building, you must also make absolutely sure that you can find your way to the correct room. Shrewd candidates also make careful note of the nearest toilets.

## WHAT TO WEAR

Clothing for an interview is largely a matter of personal choice but nevertheless the concept of 'power dressing' should be adhered to as far as possible. Whatever you select from your wardrobe your goal must be to look entirely professional and 101% appropriate for the post for which you are applying. Most senior hospital physicians are relatively conservative people in the way they dress and they will expect you to do likewise. For men a dark suit with a pristine white shirt and contrasting tie is undoubtedly the most appropriate. Your shoes must be gleaming. Men should not wear any obvious jewellery simply because it runs the risk of alienating one or more members of the panel. You may, of course, wear a discreet tie clip and appropriate, unobtrusive cuff links.

The choice of tie for men can be all important. Indeed, if you are forced into the 'uniform' of a dark suit and a white shirt, then the choice of a good tie is one of the few ways in which you can display some individuality. The tie should be of a pattern best described as 'classic'. For example, woven silk or plain silk with a simple pattern. Sometimes relatively bright colours including red, orange and bright yellow can look quite striking and yet, at the same time, retain a feeling of great professionalism. I would urge caution against wearing any sort of club tie. Even if you happen to know that the head of department was in the same Royal Air Force squadron as your father, it is ill-advised to wear the appropriate club or regimental tie since you run the risk of being questioned about the tie and its significance. One of two things will then happen: either you will be able to answer in a very erudite manner impressing the former Group Captain on the interview panel, and this will alienate the other members of the panel; or, alternatively, you will not be able to answer the probing questions relating to the provenance of your tie and you will then look totally ridiculous. Club ties, therefore, are out.

Clothing for women is altogether more difficult and it is quite reasonable to ask for advice from senior female medical colleagues. You must, of course, aim to look smart, and the goal should be to look stylish and not 'frumpy' or 'tarty'. You should ensure that you choose clothing you feel comfortable in, which you can walk in and which you can sit down safely in! Either trousers or a skirt are acceptable as long as they are smart. Whatever you choose, remember all the time that the guiding principle must be to appear totally professional. And remember to take a second pair of tights with you on the day; the pair that you are wearing when you leave home will inevitably be laddered when they get caught on the taxi door as you arrive at the interview!

One word on smell, and that is 'don't'. Excessive use of any cosmetics is to be avoided. Female candidates may, of course, risk a modest splash of perfume and apply make-up, but make-up should be done in a manner that gives a professional air without looking garish. Small items of jewellery are also quite reasonable for women. In the same way that men should avoid jewellery, men should also avoid anything other than minimal application of aftershave. Most panels will object to what they perceive as a 'man wearing perfume.'

## HOW TO SIT

It is possible to anticipate what will happen when you are called into the interview room. You will be sitting outside the room, usually with other candidates who will mostly not be engaging in conversation with you. When your name is called you need to stand up smartly and follow the invitation to enter the interview room. First impressions are all important and you need, as you go through the door, first to look professional, secondly to look interested in what is going on and thirdly — and above all — to start giving an immediate impression that you are the only suitable candidate for the job. One way to achieve this is to acknowledge as many of the interview panel as is possible at least with eye contact and perhaps a small nod. If the panel is very large this will not be possible. Do not look at the floor or stare blankly at the wall behind the chairman of the panel. Do not sit down until you are invited to do so.

If somebody — probably the chairman — shakes your hand, then try to meet his handshake with one of equal force. Don't counter his firm grasp with a limp-wristed effort, and if he is a rather frail individual with a gentle touch, do not assume that crushing his metacarpo-phalangeal joints with a vigorous response will win you any friends. If you happen to be a member of any curious societies who use a characteristic 'secret' handshake, then do *not* use it in the interview. Either it will go unnoticed and so will be of no benefit, or, in the unlikely event that the recipient of your handshake is a member of the same mysterious society, it might be perceived as a feeble effort to gain an unfair advantage in the proceedings, and this will act against you.

When you do sit, try and avoid giving the impression of a captured soldier undergoing interrogation. It is reasonable to turn the chair to a slight angle and to sit with your legs crossed if you wish with your hands on your lap. Try to avoid looking terrified or gripping the arms of the chair tightly. Do not, under any circumstances, adopt a posture that could be regarded as 'slouching'. If the chair is a relatively comfy chair with a low back, sometimes this can be difficult, and you may wish to sit forward on the edge of the chair. The overriding goal is to give an air of cool professionalism.

# EYE CONTACT, WHERE TO LOOK AND THE 'CV RUN-THROUGH'

Virtually all medical job interviews begin the same way, and that is the chairman of the panel will introduce you to all the other members of the panel. Frequently, you will know these individuals since you may have been working with them already or you may have recently had lengthy discussions with them regarding the reasons why you want this job. No matter how well you know the panel you must 'play a straight bat' from this point onwards. It may be the case that somebody interviewing you is one of your regular drinking or mountaineering partners but that fact will not be known to other members of the panel, and excessive informality simply goes down very badly. An interview is a formal occasion and you must behave appropriately. Therefore, when each member of the panel is introduced it is reasonable to nod and say, 'hello', but probably no more than that. Once the introductions are completed the chairman of the interview panel will almost certainly hand straight over to the representative of the Royal College or the national panellist, or, alternatively, another member of the panel who will start going through your CV.

Bear in mind at this point that although every word of your CV is known to you and you may be able to recite it verbatim, it is possible that the panel member now holding your CV may never have seen it before. So, although you may think it is obvious that your career progression during the past 6 years is written down with impeccable clarity, the person now looking at your hieroglyphics may not find it quite so clear. You need to nod and make small comments of agreement as this panel member starts going through your CV noting where you went to school, where you trained, where you did your house jobs, where you did your SHO rotation and so on.

While this panel member is doing this task he is totting up in his head the number of months you have spent in each job, basically satisfying himself that you have done the right amount of previous training to be suitable for the present post. Frequently, this adding up procedure goes wrong and it is perfectly reasonable for you to politely interrupt and correct the panel member if his sums are going awry. Be ready at this point to have answers to questions regarding what you did during any obvious gaps in your professional training. You may think that your CV clearly indicates the 4 months that you spent at a mission hospital in central Africa, but it may not be immediately evident to the Royal College representative struggling to find his way around your CV, and you need to be ready to help if necessary. Try to avoid getting into lengthy discussions regarding what you have or have not done in the past at this point, since this early part of the interview is very much an assessment to check that you are suitable for the job in question. Also, be absolutely certain that you can recall every detail of your own training progression since candidates who struggle to remember exactly where they did their first SHO job can look very silly indeed in front of interview panels.

Once this initial 'CV run-through' has been completed the chairman of the interview panel will invite other members of the panel to question you in turn. It is possible that not all the members of the interview panel will ask questions. The actual questions that you may be asked are dealt with in a later section of this book, but in starting to consider how to deal with the questions two general principles apply. The first of these is that whatever question you are asked you must try to give your answers promptly, brightly and using the guiding principle of 'cool professionalism with sparkle'. Your style of answering should be confident, polite, to the point and yet not bland. A brief reflective moment to gather your thoughts before you start to speak is fine, but avoid absolutely any prolonged 'pregnant pauses'. Remember that although this interview is the most important thing that has happened to you for many months, for the members of the panel it may be something of a chore and you may be the eighth candidate that they have interviewed that afternoon. Therefore, a degree of enthusiasm and sparkle must come through in all your answers to draw the attention of the panel to you and to gain their interest.

The second guiding principle for answering interview questions is related, and is this: although just one member of the panel will have asked you the question, you need to deliver your answer to all the members of the panel. In other words, although you should start by facing the questioner and beginning your answer, as you develop your reply you should engage in eye contact with other members of the panel, turning your head if necessary, to make sure that the right side of the room is not bored if the question came from the left side of the panel and vice versa. Your goal is to impress not just the person who has asked you the question but to make sure that you win over every member of the panel with every answer to every question. The art of head turning and gaining eye contact with others is not one which doctors practice. Watch politicians delivering a speech to a large audience. They do it well. That is because they have been trained, and it is quite reasonable for you to train yourself by asking some friends to give you a mock interview. If there are two or three of them make them sit in different areas of the room and practice getting all of them involved with your answers to their questions.

## GESTURE

Many interview candidates sit with their hands firmly clasped together or, worse still, their arms folded throughout the whole interview. This is a disaster and gives a very bad impression to the panel. Again, observe a politician being interviewed on television; watch how they use their hands. Seldom is there any wild, expansive gesture but very frequently there is small reinforcement of points that they are making by using small gestures with one hand. This is something that you should practice. Also, panels are very impressed with a reasoned answer containing several components, each thread of which is enumerated by tapping one finger on to the fingers of the opposite hand as though you were counting. Simple gesture makes for a good delivery and can be surprisingly good at making one candidate 'stand out from the crowd'. Gesture should be subtle and restrained but should be used. Just be careful not to overdo it to turn the whole thing into a game of charades.

## VOICE USAGE

A medical job interview is not the correct forum in which to rehearse your imitation of Richard Burton or Laurence Olivier, at least not unless your natural voice already sounds like one of them. All the same, it is worth considering before the event how you use your voice in an interview, in order to avoid disasters. For example, make sure that you do not deliver your answers like some interviewees who have an alarming tendency to drop the volume of their voice lower and lower as they speak, so that the members of the interview panel are required to lean further and further forward in their seats in order to hear what is being said.

If you have absorbed the messages given elsewhere in this book, you will know that there is a very real benefit to be gained by saying answers to 'predictable questions' out loud before the interview. Ask one of your friends to listen to you when you do so, and ask them how you sound. Most theatre and film actors will experiment many times with the manner in which they deliver a given line, and there is no reason why you should not experiment by rehearsing answers to questions in different styles beforehand. Work out which type of voice usage you feel most comfortable using.

If you feel that everything you say sounds terrible, then try sitting up straighter, opening your mouth wider, and aim to get more energy into your voice. Imagine that you have just been to the cinema and seen the best film you've seen for many years and you're describing it enthusiastically to a close friend. Think about the way you would use your voice doing that, and then use the same voice to practise delivering answers to potential interview questions. You will almost certainly sound significantly better. Remember that your goal is not just to be heard, your goal is to make an impact!

Have you ever wondered whether your *speed* of talking is correct? If so, then the answer is that it will almost certainly be too fast. If you are in any doubt at all, then *slow it down*! It is very unlikely that you will speak too slowly in the interview, but many candidates—particularly women—speak far too quickly.

## HOW TO END THE INTERVIEW

When the interview is over and all the questions have been asked then you will be invited to leave. This instruction may be preceded by the chairman of the panel letting you know that they will come to a decision perhaps later that day, in which case he may invite you to wait. Alternatively, he may suggest that the decision will not be made until the following day, in which case he will ask whether the secretary of the panel has appropriate contact details for you. Make up your mind in advance whether you are going to stay to hear the result if it is only going to be an hour or so later. In general terms interview panels like to be able to greet the successful candidate at the end of the afternoon, so stay if you can. However, if you have travelled a long distance and have a train or plane to catch to return home, then they will not be irritated if you ask them to contact you by telephone with news of the outcome.

When you stand from your chair do not blindly walk out of the room but make a point of acknowledging as many members of the panel as possible with a small nod and the single phrase, 'thank you', addressed to the panel as a whole. Then leave, trying to ensure that you know which way the door of the interview room opens to avoid unnecessary pulling when you should be pushing. You must also make absolutely certain that you do not use the wrong door and unintentionally exit into the broom cupboard, thus generating an embarrassing scene with any pretence of 'cool professionalism' being irretrievably lost.

# SPECIFIC INTERVIEW STRATEGIES

## chapter 5

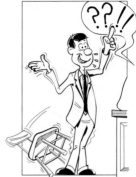

At the start of this book, I suggested that getting yourself onto the short list should be viewed as something akin to a military operation. Once you are in the interview itself, however, there is generally no need for such covert manoeuvering, and you can simply be yourself, answering questions with professionalism and enthusiasm. Sometimes, though, you may have a suspicion before the interview that you are in a certain position 'in the running', and under these circumstances it is occasionally worth modifying your approach very slightly.

## 'I'M IN THERE ALREADY'

If you really know before the event that you are the 'front runner' (and, of course, this would be a very happy position in which to be), then your biggest risk is that you somehow 'blow it'. Therefore make sure that you handle the interview in a smooth, professional, and orthodox way. By all means be animated and enthusiastic, but make sure that you don't 'overtalk' or start to deliver an unnecessary lecture mid-interview which may run the risk of alienating one or more members of the panel.

Give well-considered and thoughtful answers to questions, avoiding controversy, and keep in the back of your mind that all you have to do is *confirm* to the panel that you are the right person for the job. Do not risk losing the backing of people who may already be your main supporters by saying anything inflammatory or very unexpected, and above all do not be flippant. In other words, play the interview with a 'straight bat'.

## THE RANK OUTSIDER

The situation is different if you know that you are an outsider and way down the list of likely winners. Under these circumstances a 'straight bat' interview is fine, but is very unlikely to get you the job. Therefore you may want to risk a much more aggressive stance, and deliver a so-called 'machine gun interview'. This style of interview technique aims to leave a panel saying 'Wow!' when you leave the room, and gets your name mentioned in the consideration of the 'final few' when the panel start their deliberations.

The trick is for you to be noticeably more dynamic than all the other candidates, with imaginative and possibly even rather 'whacky' answers to questions. Some answers you give might be deliberately provocative to try to get the panel engaged in a robust discussion with you. It is also fine in this style of interviewing to offer answers to questions which many people would consider out-of-line with majority opinion on a subject, provided you can justify and expand on what you are saying. Smile a lot, really trying to engage every panel member, and try to come over as an individual with a great passion and strength of feelings about the subjects raised. The hope is that one or two members of the panel may be attracted to someone whom they feel is 'more sparky' than the rest of the field, and they might just offer you the job. Bear in mind, however, that this is a very 'high-risk' strategy, and it may well fail. So only consider this sort of approach if you know that the interview is unlikely to lead to success!

## UNORTHODOXY

With the exception of the 'machine gun interview' strategy described above, be very careful about unorthodoxy in an interview; in other words, don't be too unconventional or say things that are a long way out of line with accepted opinion. This rule extends to what you wear and how you enter and leave the room, as well as to what you say in response to questions. Some degree of 'distinguishing style' in an interview is fine, and the odd controversial answer to a question is usually okay, provided you make some acknowledgement that you realise your own view is not matched by others, and you can defend yourself if the panel picks up on what you have said. Often the attention of a panel is aroused by presentation of non-standard views and unexpected answers to questions, particularly if they are interviewing a large series of candidates. But remember that you are not there to provide an entertaining interlude for those people interviewing, you are there to get the job!

## LYING

This issue requires a very simple instruction: 'don't do it!' You may think that you can gloss over the 6-month 'unfilled gap' on your curriculum vitae that arose because you were on a course and badly failed the exam at the end of it; but if the panel question you about that period of time, then you should simply tell them what happened. Many people have mishaps and exam failures during the course of a medical career, and by and large interview panels are not too troubled by them. However they *will* be troubled—intensely—if they perceive that a candidate in an interview is lying to them, and it will undoubtedly guarantee failure. Even worse, if it were the case that a candidate claims to have a postgraduate qualification that they do not possess, then this becomes yet more serious, and is likely to threaten any further progression of that doctor's career, with involvement of the General Medical Council, other regulatory authorities and formal disciplinary procedures.

**Do not lie in interviews.**

# THE QUESTIONS

## chapter 6

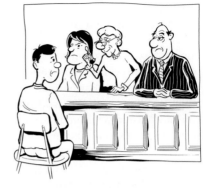

One very important mistake that interview candidates make is they fail to realise that it is entirely feasible to work out what questions you will be asked in the interview long before you ever find yourself sitting in front of the panel. Many candidates do not believe that such a feat is possible. However, the sequence of questions which is asked in a medical job interview, particularly when interviewing candidates for senior house officer (SHO) and specialist registrar posts, is remarkably consistent. To some extent the flow of questions that a candidate will be asked when applying for a consultant-grade job can also be largely anticipated in advance. In other words, some questions are inevitable.

## INEVITABLE QUESTIONS

With some thought it is very easy to see what the 'inevitable' questions will be. If, for example, you are applying to be a specialist registrar in gastroenterology in a major city in the Midlands then you will undoubtedly be asked, first, 'why gastroenterology?' and, secondly, 'why this city?' Whether you like the thought of these questions or not you are under an absolute obligation to have clear, well thought out and concise answers to both these questions. Remember, when you frame your answers that all the time the essence is not just to show that you are good at answering these questions. The overwhelming priority is to show through your answers that you are unequivocally the best person for the job. Any sort of rambling or waffling answer to these first questions, for example comments such as 'Well, I'm really not sure what I want to do, but I think gastroenterology seems like a good idea' is a recipe for disaster. Equally, when considering the city in which you have applied to work, remember that the unit in that city may have been the product of years and years of work by the members of the panel who are now interviewing you, and comments such as, 'Well, I thought I'd try here first because the advert was the first to appear in the *British Medical Journal*, but I'm equally enthusiastic about cities X and Y.' is not the sort of answer that builds up warmth between the interview panel and you.

You need to frame and construct your answers with some care, and it would be my suggestion that you adhere to the guiding principle suggested in the previous section of this book, which could loosely be described as 'cool professionalism with enthusiasm'. You must show that, first, you are perfectly capable as a doctor, secondly, that you will be capable of performing brilliantly in the post which is on offer and, thirdly, demonstrate that you are entirely professional about all you do. However, your answers must have a certain gloss—a kind of sparkle—which demonstrates an enthusiasm which is often not shown by the candidates against whom you will be competing. Therefore, let 'cool professionalism with enthusiasm' be in the back of your mind whilst you are delivering your answers.

Remember that the interview panel will like to feel that some praise is being offered for their unit through the medium of your answers. Therefore, a good answer dealing with the question 'Why do you want to come to this city?' might include observations such as: 'You have to look a long way to find a training programme in gastroenterology which is as well constructed and offers such good variety as the post in this city. There are very few other centres that allow a rotation between hospitals giving me a chance to work with a number of different consultants in the field, all of whom have differing subspeciality interests.'

You can then add other riders to your comments according to the specific circumstances of the post for which you have applied; for example, 'Of particular appeal in the present post is the close liaison which you enjoy with, (e.g.) the regional liver transplant programme, since this is an area of gastroenterology that particularly interests me.' Or you might add, for example, 'The present post is particularly exciting because of the high intensity emergency work which is done and the close links which you have with the supra-regional trauma centre which is on this site.' All the time your answers must be focused and enthusiastic making it quite plain that no other job is the one for you except for the present job which is on offer.

It is only in interviews at a relatively junior level that you can expect to be asked 'Why this subject?' and, again, your answers must be well thought out and show total enthusiasm and commitment to the speciality which you are trying to enter.

A word of caution is necessary at this point for the candidate who is applying for an SHO, specialist registrar or even consultant job in a location in which he is already working. In a previous section of this book I have drawn attention to the grave risk that candidates who are well known to the panel will be excessively informal and sometimes even flippant with an interview panel whom they already know well. This is a great mistake and is to be avoided at all costs. This scenario also gives rise to a question which may floor an unwary candidate and that is something along the lines of: 'Surely, having worked with us for the past 12 months you cannot possibly want to carry on working with us for the next 5 or 6 years?' This sometimes comes as an unexpected question for a candidate and a clear answer, again avoiding inappropriate humour or flippancy, is necessary. My suggestion would be to turn the question on its head and use it to your advantage by saying something along the lines of: 'It is precisely because I have had the opportunity of working in this department and with several members of the panel that I realise exactly what an excellent opportunity for further training in gastroenterology this unit offers. I have had the opportunity to take part in the in-patient and out-patient service as well as helping to shape our present emergency service, and I very much want to develop these aspects of the service in the next stage of my career.'

It would be perfectly reasonable to add (whether you believe it or not): 'Indeed, having had the opportunity to compare my experience in this department with colleagues who have worked in other departments, I can see that there are few other departments around the country that can offer (e.g.) a specialist registrar position with so many exciting opportunities as the present post.' And you could conclude this rather difficult moment in the interview by reinforcing the point, '. . . so it is *because* I am already familiar with the department that I am so excited and enthusiastic about the present post which is on offer.'

## PROBABLE QUESTIONS

Some of the questions that are listed above can be guaranteed to be asked in just about every medical interview. There will then follow a series of questions which can also largely be anticipated. If you are applying for a post at a junior level you will be asked about your experience of the clinical training course in your medical school, how much time you spent in general medicine, general surgery, accident and emergency and so on. Most interview panellists who will be genuinely interested in the medical curricula at other medical schools may well ask a question along the lines of: 'If you were planning your own medical curriculum what would you alter?' There is no right or wrong answer to this, but a thoughtful answer which makes sense to the interview panellist will usually go down well.

In framing an answer to this sort of a question you should be prepared to provoke a little discussion with the panel and don't worry if they seem to disagree with some of your observations; stick to your guns and say why you would change the curriculum in the way that you have proposed. The only wrong way to answer the question is to spend a long time 'umming' and 'aaahing' and then say something rather limp like, 'Well I thought our course was probably alright, I don't think anything needs changing.' This sort of answer loses the feeling of enthusiasm which you are trying to convey.

Again, if you are applying for a post at a relatively junior level you can be certain that some time will be spent asking about your elective period. Be sure that you know exactly where you went, and if you worked with anybody famous, who they were, since it is possible that they will be known to the panel. Conversely, if you went somewhere exotic, for example, the Caribbean and spent the whole 8-week period playing golf, lying on the beach and windsurfing, then do not say this in your answer. Whilst many interview panels will realise that this is a very important part of student elective periods, they will not wish to be told so in the formal environment of an interview, and you must therefore be prepared to talk about the difficulties of delivering community paediatric care in remote areas of Caribbean islands or something similar. Remember that you are showing 'cool professionalism' all the time. Whilst one or two members of the panel may, themselves, be enthusiastic golfers or windsurfers, they will not wish to hear that this was the way in which you spent your elective period.

Research and publications are a guaranteed part of any interview. If you have had the skill to produce an undergraduate publication and you are applying for a junior house officer (JHO) or SHO job, then undergraduate publications greatly impress the panel and you may be surprised to be asked about this in some detail. Therefore, you must be able to quote the title of any papers which resulted from your work and you should have preprepared a short paragraph in your head, which will explain in simple terms to individuals who are not familiar with your field, what you did and why your research was of interest. Remember at this point the 'vicar's wife' figure on the panel; in other words, remember that your answer must be intelligible to somebody who may not know any medicine at all. Sometimes interview candidates of both junior and senior level are quite incapable of explaining the nature of their research work in a simple way to people who are very experienced in medicine but not familiar with the specific area of research. If you cannot explain your own research in a simple way to an interview panel, then they will lose interest in your answer and, at the same time that they lose interest in your answer, they will also lose interest in you.

It is worth stressing a second 'guiding principle' at this point and that is many interview candidates believe that it is up to them to show that 'they are right for the job'. Curiously, this is not necessarily the overriding goal in an interview because it could be argued that everybody who has found their way onto the short list is 'right for the job'. If they were not 'right for the job' then they would not have been short listed in the first place. So, a second thought needs to be in the back of your mind as you are delivering all your answers in the interview, namely you need to show the panel that 'not only are you right for the job, *but the job is right for you at this stage in your career.*' This assertion requires a little thought but it is very true that there is often little to choose between interview candidates who have been short listed for a given post, and in the discussion which follows 'behind closed doors' after all candidates have been interviewed, a decision which may seem to be very difficult indeed can sometimes be resolved by the interview panel deciding the answer to the question: 'For which of the candidates whom we have just interviewed is this job the most appropriate at this stage in their career?' Therefore, if you—when delivering your answers—have stressed the point that not only are you the right, most appropriate person for the job, but also that the job is clearly the right way that you 'should be moving' at this stage in your career progression, then that message may hit home, and getting that point across is frequently the single best way to win over an interview panel. Panels do not like individuals that seem to be 'drifting' from one job to the next. They are far more impressed by an individual who has 'nailed their colours to the mast' and who has demonstrated a clear career direction. Part of that demonstration means that you need to show the panel that the job is right for you at this moment in time.

## PROBLEM QUESTIONS AND HOW TO ESCAPE

There are a number of 'sticky moments' which often crop up in interviews and rather surprisingly some of these can also be anticipated and a way out identified. It is often sensible to have identified the escape routes from these 'sticky' interview moments before you are faced with them in front of a formal panel. The following are some examples.

### You've done no research

Most hospital specialists need to do research. Certainly, they need to have published a few papers before getting to senior level. Some individuals are wonderful clinicians and seem to get a long way up the career ladder without doing any research at all. The time this matters is when they are faced with an interview panel. If your CV is short on publications and original research, then you need to have some sort of an answer ready in case this issue is brought up. Rather than meekly admitting that you are a failure when it comes to writing papers, it is better to try and turn this shortcoming into a strength, perhaps by saying something like: 'You will see from my CV that my greatest strengths are in the field of clinical medicine. My whole career so far has been very much orientated towards a clinical progression rather than a research or academic approach. I think my greatest contribution has been in liaison with my research colleagues and providing a source of patients and clinical ideas to enhance their own research. Therefore, I feel I have contributed to a number of different research projects over the years, but *as a clinician*, and I have not been the major author of any of the resulting publications.' This may or may not be true but an answer along these lines is at least an attempt to turn a weakness into a strength.

### You're applying for a 5-year rotation but the whole panel knows that you really want to go and work in Australia as soon as possible

Many junior doctors express enthusiasm to spend 1 or 2 years abroad at some point during their career and there is no need to hide this fact during the interview. The concern that worries interview panels most is if they think a new appointee is going to leave within a few months of arriving in a post since then a replacement will need to be found very quickly, and that does not go down well. You do not, however, need to keep the fact that you are thinking of doing a year or two abroad a secret, but it is reasonable to give your overseas intentions a rather low profile, and to take an approach along the lines of: 'Although I have said for some time I would be interested in exploring the possibility of working overseas for a year or two, my major interest is to get an excellent training (e.g.) in gastroenterology, and the present post offers me the chance of getting such a training. Therefore, my prime enthusiasm is to gain appointment to the present job and work my way through this rotation for a number of years. It may be in years to come I may think about exploring the possibility of a year abroad, but that would only be with the full agreement of the senior colleagues with whom I was working at that time.'

### You don't really want the job but your boyfriend / girlfriend / wife / husband works in this city

Candidates are often surprised that interview panels are remarkably human. Therefore, if you have pressing social, domestic or family reasons why you want to work in this city, then it is quite acceptable to say so. If you are a total 'no-hoper', then a plea that your boyfriend or girlfriend lives and works in this city is unlikely to secure you the job. However, if you are running neck and neck with one of the other candidates and you have a pressing domestic reason why you would like to come to this particular city, then that is often influential when it comes to decision time. Accordingly, you do not need to be afraid of mentioning your social situation as one reason for wanting to work in a particular city. Comments in that regard, however, *must* be linked with the sorts of answers offered in paragraphs above, indicating a strong enthusiasm for the post, the training that is offered, the individuals with whom you would be working and so on.

### It's far too early in your career for the job that you are applying for but you are 'chancing your arm'

This is a difficult issue and interview panels will often identify this problem very quickly. Occasionally, extreme enthusiasm and confidence both before and during the interview will win the day here. This problem is actually less frequent following the introduction of the Calman training system for specialist registrars in the UK, since this system now dictates that candidates must have done a certain amount of general professional training or 'GPT' at SHO level before they are allowed to enter the specialist registrar grade, and at the end of the specialist registrar period there is a strictly-defined time period during which specialist registrars may start to look for their consultant job.

Nevertheless, it sometimes happens that a relatively junior SHO wants to apply for the perfect specialist registrar rotation in the very best centre, and, in my view, it is quite reasonable to make every effort to get that job since the chance may not come around again for very many years. You must then be prepared to take a relatively aggressive stance in an interview making it quite plain that you feel very confident in your ability to perform well in the job for which you are applying. You need to show that you have masses of experience in the short time that you have been an SHO and that you have made a great effort to get to know the new hospital, unit and ward in which you will be working. You need to stress repeatedly during your answers that you feel 'entirely confident that you would be able to perform the job appropriately', but bear in mind your answers must not be so aggressive as to sound 'cocky' or over-confident. If you really feel that the present post is the chance of a lifetime then by all means say so in the interview, since this will continue the air of *professionalism with enthusiasm*, which is so important in ensuring success.

## You're really not sure if you want this job or not

This is an issue that I addressed in the first section of this book. There is simply no excuse for sitting in an interview for a job which you are not totally certain that you want. Of course, you *may* apply for a job and then withdraw prior to the interview. Even if you find yourself in the horrible situation that you are in front of the interview panel and then decide that you really do not want the job, then you should say so and explain your reasons why. The real catastrophe is when individuals do well in an interview, are offered the job, and then decline the job a couple of days—or worse still—a couple of weeks later. This generates intense animosity on the part of interview panels who will then have to be reconvened in order to appoint another candidate. It will potentially wreck your career because word gets around that you have 'dropped out after appointment' and there is certainly a chance that your referees will be contacted and an explanation will be demanded as to why you have behaved in the way that you have. Therefore, if you are not certain that you want this job make sure that you are not in the interview in the first place!

## 'CRINGE' QUESTIONS

Medical interviews are different from many other sorts of interview. Some people see them as more challenging than the interviews which our colleagues in industry face; others see them as very much lighter than the gruelling interviews faced by professionals in other walks of life. For example, if you were being interviewed for a post outside the world of medicine you might find yourself being asked a series of rather curious questions, for example: 'What are your strengths?', 'What are your weaknesses?', 'What was your greatest achievement?'. These are questions which most medical students and doctors would not find easy to answer at the best of times, and they sometimes, albeit infrequently, crop up in medical interviews. They usually come from a panel member who cannot think of anything better to ask, and occasionally they come from the 'vicar's wife' figure on the panel. These are sometimes rather irreverently referred to as 'cringe questions'. They gain that name because not only will you cringe when the question is posed, but virtually every other member of the interview panel will also inwardly cringe with embarrassment. So you need to get through these questions as quickly as possible, whilst at the same time not saying anything incriminating. Most of us could offer a fair answer to the question 'What are your strengths?' and an answer such as: 'I'm a hard worker, I'm enthusiastic in what I do, and most people say that I am very easy to get on with.' is perfectly adequate, and is quite long enough.

Rather harder is framing an answer to the question: 'What are your weaknesses?' On occasion I have heard candidates offer astonishingly foolish answers to this question which immediately exclude them from any chance of success in the interview. For example, statements such as: 'Well, sometimes I find it impossible to get out of bed in the morning', or worse still: 'Well, I think I have a tendency to upset the nursing staff on my ward', reveal commendable frankness but are catastrophic in terms of securing success in the interview. I suggest that the only suitable answer for the 'weakness' question needs to be something that allows the rest of the panel to chuckle and get over their embarrassment quickly. A good answer might be: 'I must admit that I am obsessively punctual and completely intolerant of sloth', ideally delivered with a wry smile around the table. This sort of thing allows everybody on the panel to relax again.

As regards your 'greatest achievement', then few of us would feel that anything that we have done in medicine really rates as 'our greatest achievement'. If, however, you singlehandedly ran a paediatric surgical unit in the middle of rural Africa during your student elective period, then it might be reasonable to say so at this point. If you do not have an obvious medical achievement which is breathtaking, it is often better to retreat to a rather endearing answer and reply with something like: 'Being awarded my 50 metres swimming certificate at the age of 5.' or 'Receiving an invitation to give a solo organ recital in the local cathedral, following a successful school concert.'

## 'GOOGLIES'

Sometimes an interview panel member will throw a very unexpected and rather difficult question at you. It may be a confusing question or may seem to be needlessly aggressive. They are doing this for a reason, and that is simply to see whether you are able to spark and cope when put under a bit of pressure. These questions are sometimes referred to as 'googlies'. It does not happen very often but you need to be prepared for the sort of question that goes: 'I see that you have just spent 6 months working in Sunnydale Accident and Emergency unit. Everybody knows that that unit is totally useless and should be closed down forthwith. Don't you agree?' Remember that the other interview panellists will be surprised at hearing a question like this from one of their colleagues, and therefore this can work to your favour. The interest of the interview panel will suddenly have been aroused and you can maintain their interest by being equally robust in your answer which might be along the lines of: 'No, I totally disagree. I am aware of the rumours circulating regarding the Sunnydale casualty service but having worked there very recently I find these stories astonishing. They are totally unfounded. Furthermore, I would suggest that some of the work practices which we employ at Sunnydale are streets ahead of the services offered at comparable units. I think that the people making these criticisms should come and spend some time with us and see exactly what they could learn from the set-up at Sunnydale.'

You may get other questions that are less aggressive but equally likely to fox the unwary candidate. For example: 'If the centre of Birmingham were hit by a nuclear bomb tomorrow and all the hospitals at which you have been working during the past 5 years were destroyed, how would you rebuild them? Would it be one huge hospital or several small ones?' Obviously, there is no right or wrong answer to this sort of question but panels will be genuinely interested in your view. Any sort of well thought out plan to redevelop health services in Birmingham would be an acceptable answer. A bad answer would be something along the lines of: 'Well, I don't really know—I've never really put much thought into how hospitals function. I wouldn't be able to plan for a project like that.' This sort of feeble answer lacks enthusiasm and lacks sparkle.

## HANDLING THE 'VICAR'S WIFE' PANEL MEMBER

You may well be asked questions by the lay member of the panel. It is an unfortunate fact that most of the other members of the interview panel will be rather less interested in the questions that come to you from this individual, and probably less interested in your answers. Therefore, your answers need to be polite, enthusiastic but very much to the point. For example, if it says on your CV that you write children's books in Welsh then it is almost a running certainty that the lay member of the panel will want to spend some time talking to you about this. You need to be focused and crisp in your answers. This is because although it may be of great personal interest to you that you have achieved such literary success in Wales, it will not, however, be of any great interest to the rest of the interview panel. Your answers will give little clue as to whether you are or are not capable of doing the medical job for which you have applied. So you need to smile, be polite, but keep your answers relatively short when it comes to the lay member of the panel. Remember all the time that you are trying to show cool professionalism with enthusiasm and that 'cool professionalism' means professionalism as a medic not as a children's author. In your answers aim to keep coming back to your great enthusiasm for the medical subject for which you are applying. Avoid at all costs starting giving a mini-lecture on a non-medical subject to which you devote your spare time.

## HILL WALKING AND MOTORBIKES

On your CV there will be a section headed 'interests', and towards the end of the interview one or other member of the panel will ask you something about your hobbies. The guiding principle here is similar to the principle which must be adopted when handling the 'vicar's wife' in that you need to be aware that there is a risk of becoming involved in a rather lengthy, and inappropriate, discussion on diverse aspects of hill climbing, mountaineering equipment and so on. This may be of interest to the odd member of the panel who knows something about the sport, but will be of virtually no interest to any other member of the panel, all of whom will be getting bored at this stage in the interview. Therefore, if you are an enthusiastic hill walker or motorcyclist it is perfectly reasonable to say so, perhaps commenting in a sentence or two on the problems faced by the British motorcycle industry in the face of competition from the Japanese. However, do not get bogged down in this, since that it is not what you are in a medical interview for. You can save that sort of discussion for the celebratory beer once you are successful after the interview.

## 'ANY QUESTIONS FOR THE PANEL . . .?'

In the same way that you can predict the opening questions in a medical interview, you can guarantee what the final question will be. The chairman of the panel will look at his colleagues and then will turn to you and will say something along the lines of: 'Well, that is all the questions we have for you. I wonder if you have any questions for us?' What, in fact, the chairman of the panel is saying is that in their opinion the panel feel that the interview is now at an end. They wish to see the back of you and start on the next candidate. All of them are probably hoping that you will *not* have 'any questions for the panel.' Moreover, if you do have questions that you want to put to the panel now is not the right time to do it. You should have done it before the interview, and if you have overlooked anything then you should sort it out afterwards.

I suggest, therefore, that there is only one suitable answer to this question and that is something along the lines of: 'Thank you, but no. I have had the chance of meeting several members of the panel in advance of this interview and all my questions have been answered. Thank you.' And at that point you shut up. Somebody will then stand up and show you the way to the door. That is the time to leave.

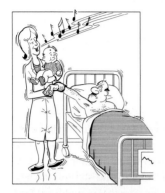

# POTENTIAL MINEFIELDS FOR WOMEN CANDIDATES

## chapter 7

## CAREER GAPS TO HAVE CHILDREN

Like it or not, there can be specific problems that women candidates will face in a medical job interview. Historically, hospital consultants have tended to be male and often quite conservative in their outlook. Most members — and certainly the chairman — of an interview panel are now acutely aware that there are significant restrictions on the the type of questions that can be asked of a female candidate, and all would agree that questions such as, 'Are you thinking of leaving 6 months after appointment to have children?' are both unacceptable and outrageous. Nevertheless, the fact that your curriculum vitae shows that you have already had a year or two off in order to have children may, no matter how inappropriately, be brought up during the interview.

With a little forethought, troublesome questions like these can be turned to your advantage. It is entirely reasonable to explain to an interview panel that your two main priorities in life are, first, your family and, secondly, your career. And stress to the panel that the priorities *go in that order*. Most interview panels would have to agree that there is 'never a right time' in the ascent of the hospital doctor career ladder to have children, and the majority will be impressed by someone who has managed to juggle pregnancy, babies, young children and a career as a junior hospital doctor.

You may be able to make light of an inappropriate question and 'spin' the answer to your advantage. For example, you might comment that you have benefited from experience of sleepless nights and now have 'great experience in dealing with vomiting'. You could observe that unlike other members of the panel you have now—perhaps—been a patient yourself and have come to realise what it is like waiting a prolonged period of time for an out-patient appointment, or worse still waiting several hours before an anaesthetist came to give you an epidural. You might move on to say that your experience as a pregnant mother has given you rare insights into some of the more irritating aspects of hospital practice such as being dealt with by a doctors and nurses who fail to introduce themselves.

In general terms, even the most fuddy-duddy consultants on an interview panel are now realising that the 'work–life balance' is important today, and they will respect somebody who is able to talk about it authoritatively during a formal interview. So the main message here is: if the panel tries to attack you with an inappropriate or outrageous question make sure that you 'come out fighting' and hit back hard at them.

## APPLYING FOR A JOB SHARE

The concept of the 'job share' is not new. In many walks of life, particularly in industry and the Civil Service, job sharing is now commonplace. Unfortunately, it is observed less frequently in day-to-day hospital practice. There is no good reason for this, and if you feel that the most appropriate next move on the career ladder is to a post that is shared with another individual then do not hesitate to apply for such a position. More importantly, be aware that a post that is advertised as a full-time job can often be performed highly effectively by two people job sharing, so be prepared to go and speak to the relevant consultants and human resources department to suggest that a full-time job which they have just advertised could perhaps be filled by means of a job share.

The key point that needs to be considered when applying for a job share post in a hospital is whether to apply in the hope that another like-minded individual will also apply to make up the 'other half' of the job share, or whether you should apply with a 'ready-made partner' and present yourselves as a unit of two people in the interview. If at all possible, I would suggest that the latter approach is the better of the two. If you enter an interview seeking to work in a job-share post and make it plain that you're already on good terms with the other doctor applying, then you will be well placed to counter any anxieties on the part of the panel regarding logistics and communication between the two doctors who would fulfil a single role. A panel may, for example, ask what you would do if your child became ill during one of the days when you should be working in hospital. The fact that you knew your job-share partner in advance of the interview would then allow you to say that you had already made contingency plans for such eventualities. They may well ask how you would communicate about your patients, and you should explain that you would follow a standard professional 'hand over' procedure as used by all other doctors. Your goal must be to reassure the panel that you and your job-sharing partner would fill the post on offer with as much, if not greater, reliability than a single person.

## OTHER DELAYS IN CAREER PROGRESS

There are a number of other reasons, not necessarily specific to female candidates, for an apparent delay in an individual's career progression which may alarm members of an interview panel. Examples would include time taken off in order to look after elderly parents, time spent abroad accompanying a partner on a sabbatical or other overseas placement, and perhaps time spent doing a prolonged adventurous activity such as a year-long round-the-world yacht race. The art of dealing with these issues during a job interview is to make sure that you are not pushed into viewing these periods of time as any sort of a negative experience; rather you should present them as a positive experience which sets you apart from the other candidates. You will need to stress that although your medical career inevitably was put on hold as a result of these activities, you have gained in so many other ways, be they cultural, linguistic, or simply by gaining an in-depth experience of the 'receiving end' of the National Health Service.

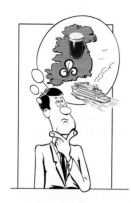

# ACTUAL QUESTIONS AND ANSWERS

**chapter 8**

## GOOD, BAD AND GHASTLY

In an ideal world, a book such as this giving guidance on inter-view technique would include a computerised CD-ROM which would contain recordings of questions asked and the answers given, in a genuine interview situation. Unfortunately, price and strict rules regarding the confidentiality of what is said during an interview, prevent such an inclusion. Nevertheless, in the para-graphs which follow I have presented a few examples of actual questions asked, and the answers given by candidates, heard by myself and some of my colleagues in medical job interviews. These are not, strictly speaking, word-for-word reproductions of what was said, and in most instances I have slightly changed the form of words used in order to preserve confidentiality, but these examples are illustrative.

It will be appreciated that many of these questions fall into the categories of 'cringe questions' and 'googlies' referred to in an earlier chapter. I've made some comments after each one.

Questioner (in a consultant interview): 'Looking at your CV, I would say that you'd be far more suited to a career in research and academia. Why you are applying for a full-time NHS post?'

Candidate (unsuccessful): 'Research is too much like hard work in my view.'

This answer fell into the category of excessive and inappropriate honesty together with a degree of flippancy. A priority in any medical interview is the recognition that it is a formal situation, and particularly in in a consultant level interview, jocularity in dealing with a question like this was not appropriate. With a little thought, the candidate could have framed a far more impressive and reasonable answer.

Questioner (specialist registrar interview): 'I'd like you to choose one adjective that describes yourself. What is it?'

Candidate (successful): 'Approachable.'

This was undoubtedly a 'cringe question', and most members of the panel gave a small intake of breath when it was asked. Nevertheless, it seems to be a question which is relatively frequently used both in medical interviews and elsewhere. The answer that the successful candidate gave was a good one, because it was novel and thoughtful, and it followed a series of weaker answers from other candidates, including predictable ones such as 'enthusiastic', 'keen' and 'friendly', and the dreadful answer 'Gosh, that's difficult, I can't think of anything.'

Questioner (specialist registrar interview): 'I'd like you to pick one paper which you have recently read in a medical journal. Tell me about it.'

Candidate (unsuccessful): 'I can't think of one.'

This question fell into the category of 'predictable questions', and the answer was unforgivable. Every candidate for a hospital doctor post should at least have some idea of what has appeared in the medical journals in the weeks prior to their interview. Even if the candidate had not been able to comment on a specific scientific paper, he could at least have discussed an interesting editorial in one of the medical journals or, if all else failed, steered the question to talking about a medical piece in the national press.

Questioner (in an specialist registrar interview, to an Irish doctor): 'I see that you're Irish, and you trained in Ireland. Isn't it a well-known fact that all Irish graduates inevitably return to Ireland in the long run, so why should we give you postgraduate training here?'

Candidate (successful): 'That's not true at all! Whilst it may be the case that many Irish doctors who have been SHOs in Ireland come to Britain for a while and then go back straight after their registrar post, you'll see from my CV that I left Ireland as a JHO and have worked in the United Kingdom ever since then. I have every intention of remaining in Britain for the foreseeable future and when I eventually apply for my consultant post I'll make a decision at that stage whether I want to stay in Britain or go back to Ireland.'

This question could be classed as a 'googly'. The questioner was presumably being deliberately provocative to see how the candidate reacted. It was a robust, fair and sensible answer.

Questioner (in a research registrar interview): 'Do you think that all hospital doctors should spend a period of time in research?'

Candidate (successful): 'No. I have a large number of colleagues who aim to become hospital consultants. Some of them are obviously well-suited to research whereas others are not. Some of these others would be far better placed, and of more use to their eventual employer, if they spent a period of time gaining, for example, an MBA degree. I think there probably should be more alternatives in the medical career ladder to the traditional 2 or 3-year period of research.'

There was no right or wrong answer to this question. The candidate said what he thought and presented his views well.

Questioner (in a specialist registrar interview where two posts at two different centres were on offer): 'You know that there are two posts on offer at the moment. I see that you have only applied for one of them. What's wrong with the post at my hospital?'

Candidate (successful): 'Of course there is nothing wrong with the post at your hospital, and all things being equal I would have applied for both posts. Unfortunately, if I were appointed to the post in your centre, I would be geographically disadvantaged, because my boyfriend lives in the other city.'

The questioner presented this question in a slightly cheeky way. The candidate responded in similar vein and generated some humour among the interview panel when she used the phrase 'geographically disadvantaged'. It was a perfectly reasonable explanation for why she had applied for only one of the two posts on offer.

Questioner (specialist registrar interview): 'There are six candidates for this job sitting outside the door, all of whom have similar CVs. Why should we have you?'

Candidate (unsuccessful): 'Well, err . . . I suppose I get on okay with people, I'm reliable and will do the work. Otherwise I don't really know.'

The answer to this question began fairly badly and then got even worse. A question like this demands a punchy, well-prepared and unequivocal answer that leaves the panel no option other than to appoint. In this example, the candidate began in a slightly self-effacing manner, and then ended extremely limply. All candidates should have a powerful ready response to this question to show the panel why they are 'the best'.

Questioner (senior house officer interview): 'I see that you've just taken 12 months off for a round-the-world yacht race. Surely that was a complete waste of time?'

Candidate (successful): 'In the past 12 months I've learnt a fantastic range of skills. Specifically, I've learnt how to work in a team and I've learnt a great deal about man management. I've also had to keep my head in extremely testing and demanding situations where there was potential for catastrophe if things went wrong. I'm certain that skills like these can only help the progress of my medical career.'

Once again, this was a slightly provocative question and the candidate handled it extremely well. She made some powerful points in her answer and this impressed the panel.

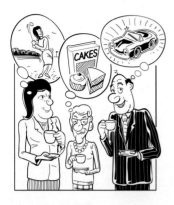

# WHAT HAPPENS BEHIND THE SCENES?

**chapter 9**

## WHO CHOOSES THE PANEL AND HOW ARE PANEL MEMBERS SELECTED?

The composition of the interview panel will vary according to the grade of post for which you are applying. It is not unknown for junior house officer (JHO) and stand-alone senior house officer (SHO) appointments to be made by a couple of consultants rather hastily grabbed on the day of the interview, or possibly asked if they are able to interview just the day before. Things are usually more formalised for appointments to an SHO rotation, for specialist registrar posts, and are very much more rigid for appointments at consultant level. For hospital training posts it is generally the local postgraduate medical department that will take responsibility for convening the panel. In contrast, if the appointment is for a consultant post then the hospital management will almost certainly take on that duty, and it will usually be the director of human resources who is responsible for the selection of panel members.

In the earlier sections of this book I have mentioned the requirement for certain individuals to be on the interview panel, particularly for appointments at specialist registrar and consultant level.

These are the representatives of the relevant Royal College in England and Wales, or 'national panellists' in Scotland. For each medical speciality in every health region there are often only a few individuals who are able to fulfil the role of Royal College representative and therefore the date of interview and the selection of the other members of the interview panel are often determined by the availability of the appropriate college representative or national panellist. Personnel departments that are trying to set up an interview will usually contact the Royal College representative first and, once they have secured their availability for a specific date, then the other members of the panel are chosen. Usually human resources departments find that they have relatively little choice in the availability of other consultants to act as members of an interview panel, because of clinical and teaching commitments as well as other engagements. However, for some posts, particularly at consultant level, there is a minimum number of individuals who are required to be on an interview panel in order for it to be 'quorate', and, accordingly, consultants may sometimes be plucked out of their clinical work to sit on a panel at very short notice indeed. As a result, the group of consultants who find their way onto an interview panel is often something of a random selection.

## WHO IS THE CHAIRMAN?

The chairman of an interview panel—particularly for consultant grade appointments—is usually a senior consultant from a speciality which is *not* the one to which an appointment is being made. The main role of the chairman is to ensure 'fair play', and therefore there is some merit in that individual not being a close colleague of the other members of the panel, almost all of whom *will* be specialists in the relevant discipline. This rule does not hold true for junior appointments, for example to an SHO rotation, when the chairman of the panel could simply be one of the assembled team of physicians or surgeons selected at the start of the interview by his colleagues. It is important to note that, strictly speaking, the chairman of the interview panel is a non-voting member. They do, however, take responsibility for collating the votes of members of the panel at the end of the interview process, and in the event of a tie, they would almost certainly be obliged to make a 'casting vote'.

## WHAT ARE THEY TOLD BEFOREHAND?

The interview panel will usually be asked to attend the interview room some 15–20 minutes before the arrival of the first candidate. If the chairman of the panel is good at his job, then a semi-formal briefing of the other panel members will take place. The chairman will ensure that all members of the panel have been introduced to each other and that they appreciate who is the Royal College representative. He will remind the panel members what the post is that they are about to appoint, he will instruct them that all discussion within the interview room is confidential and he will also ensure that none of the panel members has any 'conflict of interest' in the interview process. This latter point may present a problem in interviews for appointments to small specialities, for example if several local specialist registrars are applying for a consultant post in their own hospital. Under these circumstances it is very probable that some of the local consultants may be on friendly terms with the specialist registrars and, if that is the case, there is a requirement—at least in theory—that panel members declare it. Such an announcement does not, however, preclude a consultant's ability to remain on the panel: the chairman will simply make note of what has been said and confirm with the remaining members of the panel that they do not consider it to be a problem.

In recent years, there has been one significant change in the instructions given to interview panel members, and many of them find this rather irritating. Namely, the chairman of the panel will advise them that they should address *the same question to each can-*

*didate* who is interviewed. The logic behind this new development is understandable, as it removes one potential variable in the interview process, and arguably leads to a fairer outcome. Unfortunately, most panel members do not like this instruction, since they would prefer to ask different questions according to the background and experience of the candidate whom they are interviewing, and often want to frame their questions in reaction to answers which have been given by the interviewee up to that point. Frustratingly, it is not possible to know in advance of your own interview whether you will receive exactly the same set of questions as all the candidates who have been interviewed before you, but this is now certainly a possibility.

## WHAT DO THEY DISCUSS WHEN YOU'VE GONE?

When the final interview candidate has left the room, the chairman of the interview panel will usually look around, smile at his colleagues, and say: 'Right, who's for coffee?' There then follows 5 minutes of relaxed discussion, usually relating either to golf or to the most recent model of convertible Mercedes. This happy diversion is eventually brought to a close by the chairman who will attempt to 'bring the panel to order', and will remind the panel members that there is some 'work to do'.

The precise sequence of what happens next varies from panel to panel and is generally determined by the chairman. Typically the chairman of the panel will turn to the Royal College representative and will ask whether all the candidates are suitable for appointment or not. It is very unusual for the Royal College representative to find that one or more individuals cannot be appointed for some reason, but should that be the case, then this is the point at which they will say so. The excluded candidate or candidates will not be considered any further during the selection process.

Once this particular formality is over, every other member of the interview panel will then be invited to say a few words about the various applicants. In general terms most panel members will conclude their comments by suggesting their preferred 'one, two, three'. In other words, this is the stage during the interview process when each panel member makes a suggestion as to which candidate, they think, is the most appropriate, who is second best and who is third best. The chairman of the panel will take responsibility for collating these observations made by panel members. Usually, he will record these views on a formal 'voting grid', marking '1', '2', '3' and so on, alongside each candidate's name. Surprisingly, there is often broad agreement between panel members as to which are the three or four best candidates, and the same names are heard in each member's summary of their views. If this is the case, then the chairman simply looks at his grid and may be able to make an immediate announcement as to which is the successful candidate based on what he has heard so far, i.e. he can add up the numbers on the grid in front of him, and the candidate with the *lowest* score will be the first to be appointed, *provided that that candidate gained a vote from every panel member*. In the same way—if several appointments are being made, for example, to a number of SHO posts—the chairman will be able to use the scoring grid in order to work out which candidate has come second, which third, up to the required number of appointees for the posts on offer.

Sometimes the chairman will instruct the interview panel to consider the candidates in a different way. Rather than asking for votes, he may suggest that the panel has a general discussion, to see if there are any candidates who have just been interviewed who are clearly not going to be in the top three or four. Again, if there is agreement between the interview panel, then these names will be deleted and excluded from further discussion. This mechanism then leaves the panel with just three or four names to consider, and further discussion will then ensue with the chairman finally asking the panel to remove another one or two names, leaving final consideration of — perhaps — just the top two. There will then be a similar voting process, except all members of the panel will simply be asked to say who is their 'number one' and who is their 'number two'. In this way, a clear decision is usually reached.

Obviously these systems are not universal, and often a different strategy is needed if a large number of posts are being appointed, for example to an SHO rotation in a major teaching hospital, or if there are just two candidates for a senior professorship. Nevertheless, candidates can be reassured that enormous effort goes into making sure that the appointments process is as fair as it can be, and unsuccessful candidates who come away from interviews announcing that they consider the panel was 'rigged' or that the appointment was a 'set-up' are almost invariably wrong.

## HOW IMPORTANT ARE THE REFERENCES?

Most interview candidates would be surprised to learn that the references play relatively little part in the interview process. Indeed, it is very often the case that references are not consulted until the panel has decided who are the top one or two candidates. Sometimes the final decision is made with recourse to the references taking place only as an afterthought. The main role of the reference, therefore, is as an instrument to reassure the panel that the decision which they have made on the strength of the interview is the correct one.

It is not unheard of for the panel to decide who is their preferred first choice and who their second choice, and then find something slightly untoward or possibly disturbing in the reference for the winning candidate. Under these circumstances, the chairman will usually ask the panel if they wish to reconsider the order of their 'top two', and sometimes the individual who was positioned in second place is then awarded the job. Accordingly, having top-quality references is highly important, but your references may only play a crucial part right at the very end of the interview process.

# AFTER THE INTERVIEW

## chapter 10

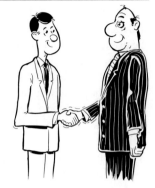

## THE JOB OFFER

If all has gone according to plan then a short while after the interview is finished the chairman of the panel will come out of the interview room and will invite you to 'come back in'. Almost always—but not absolutely inevitably—this means that you are the successful candidate and effectively means that you have got the job. Resist the urge to start hugging your fellow candidates at this stage, most of whom will suddenly feel an intense dislike towards you. Smile sweetly and try to look sympathetically towards the other candidates before smiling in a professional manner at the chairman of the interview panel and re-entering the room.

You will be invited to sit down and the chairman of the panel will announce something along the lines of: 'We are delighted to be able to offer you the job.' Strictly speaking, the chairman of the interview panel has just made a significant error of protocol, since in fact interview panels do not 'offer jobs', they simply make recommendations to the Trust Board of the hospital or to the regional postgraduate dean regarding who should be appointed. Only in exceptional circumstances, however, is the individual who is recommended by the interview panel not the person eventually selected for the job by the hospital. You should continue to retain a professional air and should thank the panel and agree that you will accept the job. A word of warning is necessary here since in the excitement of the moment it is very easy to make a mistake and announce that you will not just accept the job but readily also accept all the unsatisfactory aspects of the job which you read about in the job description but chose to ignore up until this point. You might be better placed to thank the interview panel and announce that you will, 'look forward to receiving their formal offer in the next day or two.' The reason why I advise a cagey approach at this point is that it is during the time between the interview and before formally accepting the offer of employment that you may need to negotiate certain aspects of the post. This tends to be far more important at consultant level than at senior house officer or specialist registrar level. You may now return home or, as is sometimes the case, accept an invitation go out for a beer with the interview panel, but whatever happens you can look forward to receiving a written letter offering you the job during the next few days.

## NEGOTIATION

Negotiation at this stage may be all important. Remember that this is the first stage in the job application process at which you are in a position of power. You must not abuse that power since an aggressive negotiation style will go down very badly with your future colleagues, and the worst case scenario is they will simply withdraw their offer of a job and will reconvene the panel with a view to appointing somebody different. You must, therefore, proceed with any negotiation with quiet diplomacy and tact, but at the same time, be confident about what you want to achieve.

## Salary

The most frequent source of negotiation is salary. In general terms, individuals moving up the junior hospital doctor ladder should not take a drop in salary. Some appointees have successfully argued that their new salary should be greater not just than their previous basic salary but greater than previous basic *plus* payments for additional duty hours or 'banding' supplement. Some hospitals are more easily won over on this point than others, but whatever the view of a given hospital, you should aim not to accept a drop in your annual basic salary.

The one important exception to this principle is when you move from the end of the specialist registrar ladder to consultant grade. At this point in the career ladder, there is no formal agreement to protect an individual doctor's salary and it is theoretically possible to lose out. For example, an individual on the top point of the specialist registrar scale, who was receiving a generous number of additional duty hour payments or top 'banding' rate, might find that they are appointed to the bottom increment of the consultant salary scale and subsequently find themselves on a lower salary. This should be resisted, and mindful of the unfair nature of such a move, most hospitals adopt a strategy as follows.

Individuals moving from a specialist registrar (or old-fashioned senior registrar) post into a consultant graded post will receive one incremental salary point up to a maximum of two increments on the consultant salary scale for demonstrating that they have one or more of the following attributes:

1 They are over the age of 35 years at time of appointment.
2 They hold a higher degree, i.e. MD or PhD.
3 They have been in a senior registrar appointment for more than 2 years before promotion to a consultant post.
4 They have previously worked as a locum consultant in their chosen speciality.

These four points are known as the 'unwritten rules' since they do not exist in any generally agreed form nor in any official document. They used to be applied by a large number of hospitals but *not by all*, and there is very little you can do to enforce the application of these unwritten rules, except negotiation and attempts at gentle persuasion of your future managers. Bear in mind that this issue is now much less relevant following the demise of the senior registrar grade. Nevertheless, senior specialist registrars who have been in post for several years may try to draw attention to these rules.

## The new consultant contract

At the time of this book's preparation, consultants throughout the UK are moving to a new system of contracts. Instead of a basic working week for consultants being made up of a number of periods of work called 'notional half days', contracts are being established based on an agreed job plan, the job plan comprising a number of 'programmed activities' (PAs) some of which are in 'direct patient care' i.e. clinics, operating theatre sessions, ward rounds and so on, and some of which are considered to be 'supporting professional activity' i.e. time for personal study, audit, research and teaching, etc. The precise terms and conditions of these new contracts vary slightly between appointments to consultant posts in England, Scotland and Wales.

There is a general assumption that the working week for most consultants will be based on ten programmed activities, but some consultants are being invited to accept contracts based on 11, 12 or even more 'PAs', and unlike the previous consultant contract such additional work receives additional salary. It is therefore vital that if you are being appointed to your first consultant post, you make absolutely certain you know and agree the content of your proposed job plan and exactly what remuneration it will attract. Organisations such as the British Medical Association can be extremely helpful in scrutinising a proposed offer of a contract and successful candidates should not hesitate to seek their professional advice before signing anything.

## With whom to negotiate?

Negotiation after the interview, and before taking up the offered post, is unlikely to be relevant to most junior doctors. It is, however, often important for new consultants. Discussion of salary should ideally take place with the chief executive of the hospital in which you will be working. There are very few other individuals, with the possible exception of the director of personnel, who have enough power to select the incremental start point of your new salary. You can seek the support of your new colleagues, but it is the managers who will ultimately decide. Remember that most hospital chief executives will be very willing to meet newly appointed consultants, especially so if they were not involved with the appointment process. It is entirely reasonable to request a meeting with this person very shortly after a successful interview. Issues such as salary and removal expenses may be raised at this meeting.

Negotiation about other aspects of your job can often better be done with the clinical director of your new unit or the medical director of the hospital in which you will be working. It is up to these individuals to ensure that you have an adequate office with a reasonable amount of space and also proper secretarial support. The level of secretarial support will vary from one job to the next but if you are primarily based in a single hospital, perhaps spending no more than a half or 1 day out per week, you should expect to have the services of a full-time secretary. Many hospital managers now view this as an unreasonable luxury but nevertheless it is what you should aim for.

New consultants may feel that there are other aspects of the post which they want to negotiate. For example, if you feel that the job description is totally unreasonable in its demands and expectations, then the time between the offer of the job and your formal acceptance is one possible time to negotiate. Bear in mind, however, that it is often easier and less inflammatory to actually change your pattern of work once you have been performing according to the original job description for a period of several months. Excessively pushy negotiation and obstruction prior to accepting the job offer may simply mean that your future colleagues turn against you and decide to offer the job to someone else.

## WHAT IF YOU WEREN'T SUCCESSFUL?

In my opinion there is no such thing as 'interview practice', at least not in front of a genuine panel. In the previous sections of this book I have urged that you obtain your practice in a mock interview situation with friends and colleagues. The real interview is inevitably a stressful occasion which requires a lot of investment of time and emotion if you are to be successful. Nevertheless, at times in your career you may fail to get the job that you want, and this can be extremely distressing as well as giving rise to a loss of self-confidence. Try to make the best of a bad job and use the experience of an unsuccessful interview as a sort of tool to help you be more successful next time.

Most members of an interview panel are very happy indeed to speak in general terms about reasons why you were not selected for a job. Remember, however, that the deliberations of an interview panel are totally confidential, so they will not be able to discuss specific issues relating to exactly what was said behind closed doors. All the same, most members of a panel welcome a quiet approach some days after the interview to ask perhaps: 'Were there any questions which I handled particularly badly?' or 'Was there anything on my CV which the panel felt made me unsuitable or inadequately qualified for the job?'

If you know members of the panel particularly well it is also useful to tactfully enquire whether 'they would advise you to continue using the same referees.' It is surprising how often, once prompted with a question such as this, a member of the interview panel will make a gentle suggestion that you, 'consider changing referee number two.' Act immediately if given important information such as this.

Do not immediately assume that failure in an interview is a 'black mark' on your record, neither should it be considered any form of failure. Often interview panels anguish at great length, deliberating between two and sometimes three names, all of whom they would very much like to appoint to their job and feel rather regretfully that there is only one job to offer. Sometimes one member of the panel is despatched from the interview room after the result has been announced in order to offer comfort to the unsuccessful candidates. Try not to feel particularly aggrieved if at this stage you are told it was 'within a millimetre' or 'If only we had two jobs you would have got the second one.' It is very easy to retort that 'a miss is as good as a mile', but instead you should bite your lip and be encouraged by these warm comments.

# CONCLUSION

## chapter 11

This book contains a lot of information that I believe will be useful for final-year medical students, junior doctors and also relatively senior doctors who are applying for the next post in their career progression. Bear in mind that it represents one style of dealing with a job application and the process of being interviewed. The style that I have described may not suit everybody, and if you feel that it would not suit you then do not use it. Do not try to pretend that you are someone other than yourself in the interview and do not try to answer questions in a way that seems somehow unnatural to you just because you think you are giving 'the right answers'.

Remember the important key messages stressed elsewhere in this text:

1 Make absolutely sure that you spot the advert in the first place.

2 Find out as much as you can about the interview panel before the interview.

3 Do not find yourself sitting in an interview for a job that you are not absolutely certain that you want.

4 Throughout the interview remember to try and give an impression of 'cool professionalism with enthusiasm'.

**5** Aim to show the interview panel not just that you are 'right for the job' but also that the job is right for you *at this stage in your career*.

If you are unsuccessful do not assume that there is no hope for you and that you are an abject failure. You may have been ranked a close second behind a future Nobel prize winner.

Good luck! There is always an unpredictable side to medical interviews and a degree of luck as well as a great deal of skill is needed. The author of this book cannot, of course, accept any responsibility whatsoever if things do not work out. Equally, do not blame the author if you find yourself being unexpectedly successful in obtaining jobs that you had not really intended to get!

# INDEX